Hana Hakim
Mohamed Derbel
Khouloud Feki

Physical and psychological impact of miscarriage on women

Hana Hakim
Mohamed Derbel
Khouloud Feki

Physical and psychological impact of miscarriage on women

ScienciaScripts

Imprint

Any brand names and product names mentioned in this book are subject to trademark, brand or patent protection and are trademarks or registered trademarks of their respective holders. The use of brand names, product names, common names, trade names, product descriptions etc. even without a particular marking in this work is in no way to be construed to mean that such names may be regarded as unrestricted in respect of trademark and brand protection legislation and could thus be used by anyone.

Cover image: www.ingimage.com

This book is a translation from the original published under ISBN 978-620-6-71530-6.

Publisher:
Sciencia Scripts
is a trademark of
Dodo Books Indian Ocean Ltd. and OmniScriptum S.R.L publishing group

120 High Road, East Finchley, London, N2 9ED, United Kingdom
Str. Armeneasca 28/1, office 1, Chisinau MD-2012, Republic of Moldova, Europe
Printed at: see last page
ISBN: 978-620-7-76165-4

TABLE OF CONTENTS

CHAPTER 1
INTRODUCTION

A miscarriage, also known as spontaneous abortion or unintentional termination of pregnancy, (1) is the most common cause of losing a baby during pregnancy and one of the most frequent complications in early pregnancy(2).

The most commonly accepted definition of miscarriage is that of the WHO, which considers miscarriage to be the spontaneous expulsion from the maternal body of an embryo or foetus, before it is viable, of less than 500g and/or less than 20-22 weeks gestation(3).

It is estimated that 15-20% of pregnancies end in miscarriage, and that 25% of women suffer a miscarriage in their lifetime. Approximately 23 million miscarriages occur each year worldwide, equivalent to 44 pregnancy losses every minute(4).

Most miscarriages occur during the first 14 weeks, and are known as early miscarriages(2).

These figures suggest that parents affected by miscarriage are not rare. This event has a particular impact on the lives of the couples concerned, as it heralds the start of a process of perinatal bereavement. Grief is a natural reaction to the process of loss and includes symptoms such as anger, worry, loneliness and sadness, sensitivity to noise, muscle weakness, sleep disturbances and crying(5).

Numerous studies have highlighted the harmful impact of miscarriage on women's mental health and the increased risk of depression and other mental health problems(6) .

Others have postulated that this difficult ordeal has not only psychological but also significant physical impacts (7) (8) (3).

These psychological and physical symptoms may appear immediately after the loss or may be delayed, exaggerated or apparently absent (9).

The results concerning the duration of depressive symptoms and perinatal bereavement after miscarriage are contradictory. Indeed, some studies have indicated that, for most women, symptoms resolve and are similar to those of the general population within 6 months to 1 year (10) (11) , while others have indicated that these symptoms persist long after the loss, up to 3 years (12) (13).

In addition, gender, age, perception of loss, life changes, coping styles and support systems influence the duration of bereavement. And in general, families react to loss according to their culture and religion (14).

Understanding the grief of bereaved parents is very important for the support professions in order to provide adequate care and support (15) (16).

These results raise questions about the situation in Tunisia. There is a significant lack of data in the scientific literature on perinatal bereavement and the effects of miscarriage on the mental and physical health of Tunisian women. This highlights a major gap in our understanding of these crucial issues in our society. It is essential to fill this knowledge gap in order to better support women facing such hardships and to develop appropriate interventions to meet their psychological and physical needs. This study was therefore carried out with the aim of filling this data gap and gaining a better understanding of the situation of bereaved Tunisian women.

The objectives of this research are therefore to :
- To assess levels of bereavement among women who have experienced a miscarriage.

- To describe the psychological consequences of miscarriage for Tunisian women.

- To describe the physical consequences of miscarriage for Tunisian women.
- To study variations in the mean total PGS score as a function of certain socio-demographic characteristics and certain medical and obstetric variables.

CHAPTER 2
MATERIALS AND METHODS

This chapter presents the methodological elements of the study. It begins with a description of the research design and setting, and a description of the sample, including inclusion and exclusion criteria. This is followed by a description of the measurement instruments, the data collection process and ethical considerations. The analysis plan concludes this chapter.

1 Methods :

1.1 Type of study :

We conducted a descriptive and analytical survey to meet the research objective mentioned in the first chapter.

1.2 Study location :

The data was collected in the obstetrics and gynaecology department of the Hédi Chaker University Hospital Centre (CHU) in Sfax, which includes post-partum, gynaecology, high-risk pregnancy and outpatient departments. This is an important referral centre for doctors, where Tunisian women from rural and urban areas in central and southern Tunisia are admitted. Given the time constraints and in order to speed up recruitment, the questionnaire was drawn up using the Google Forms platform so that it could be communicated via the internet, particularly in Facebook groups.

1.3 Study period :

Data collection took place from 12 February 2024 to 31 March 2024.

1.4 Study population :

The target population includes all Tunisian women who have had one or more miscarriages (spontaneous abortions) in their lifetime.

1.5 Sample :

1.5.1 Inclusion criteria :

Our survey sample included women who: a) had experienced at least one miscarriage, regardless of gestational age (early or late), in their lifetime; b) were aged 18 and over; c) were present in the research setting or able to complete the questionnaire via the Google

Forms version, during the study period mentioned above.

1.5.2 Exclusion criteria :

We excluded from the study: a) women who had undergone voluntary termination of pregnancy (IVG), b) women who had undergone therapeutic termination of pregnancy (TTP), c) women who had had an ectopic pregnancy (EP), and d) women who refused to take part in the study.

1.5.3 Sampling method :

Non-probability convenience sampling was used in this study.

1.5.4 Sample size :

Due to time constraints, we only distributed the questionnaire to 109 women who had experienced one or more miscarriages in their lifetime.

2 Equipment:

2.1 Measuring instruments :

Data were collected using a socio-demographic and clinical questionnaire (Appendix 1) and the Perinatal Grief Scale (PGS) (Appendix 2).

- **Socio-demographic and clinical data questionnaire**

The questionnaire was drawn up for the purposes of this study by ourselves, based on the specific literature on the subject. It consists of 32 closed and multiple-choice questions and is divided into six parts:
➢ The first part: is designed to identify the participants, including age, origin, marital status, level of education, employment status and socio-economic level.
➢ The second part is designed to assess health and lifestyle: height, weight, lifestyle habits (smoking, alcoholism) and personal medical history.
➢ The third part: designed to assess fertility and the characteristics of miscarriages.
➢ The fourth part is designed to assess the physical impact of miscarriage.

➢ The fifth part: assessing the psychological impact of miscarriage.

➢ The sixth part: assessment of the woman's relationship with her partner after the miscarriage.
- **Perinatal bereavement scale :**

The Perinatal **Grief Scale (PGS)** (Appendix 2) was used to measure grief reactions.
The original English version of the PGS comprises 104 elements and was developed by Potvin, Lasker and Todeter in 1989(17) .

The least relevant items were then removed from the scale, resulting in a PGS of 33 items with an alpha coefficient of 0.95. The authors validated this latest version in experiments involving 138 women aged an average of 28 years and 5 months in the United States. Eighty-two of these cases occurred between 0 and 15 weeks' gestation, 34 cases occurred after 16 weeks' gestation and before 28 weeks' gestation, and 22 cases occurred after 28 weeks' gestation (including 18 newborns)(18) .This 33-item Likert scale provides responses ranging from completely agree (1 point) to completely disagree (5 points). There are 3 subscales in the PGS (Active sadness, Difficulty adapting, Hopelessness) with 11 items each: The first dimension, also known as 'active grief', represents normal grief and includes questions about bereavement, the loss of the baby and crying related to the loss of the baby. A 5-response Likert-type rating scale provides scores ranging from 11 to 55 for the first dimension. The items related to 'active mourning' are numbers 1, 3, 5, 6, 7, 10 and 12, 13, 14, 19 and 27. The second dimension, called "Coping/Adaptation Difficulties", refers to difficulties in reconciling daily activities and family and friends, and may indicate severe depression or difficulties in functioning with family and friends. The score for this dimension varies between 11 and 55. The items related to the "coping difficulties" scale correspond to nos. 2, 4, 8, 11, 21, 24, 25, 26, 28, 30 and 33.The third dimension represents 'hopelessness' and suggests a high potential for significant and chronic effects related to the loss, such as emotional difficulties progressing to depression. The score also varies between 11 and 55. The items relating to the despair scale can be found at nos. 9, 15, 16, 17, 18, 20, 22, 23, 29, 31 and 32. Each dimension represents a different qualitative aspect of grief and a progression in the severity of grief reactions. The total score of the PGS (Perinatal Grief Scale) is obtained by first inverting all the items (i.e. scores 1, 2, 3, 4 and 5 are considered for the options of "strongly disagree", "disagree", "neither disagree nor agree", "agree", and "strongly agree", respectively), with the exception of items 11 and 33. Thus, higher scores now reflect more intense grief. The scores are then added together. The total score can vary from 33 to 165, the higher the score the greater the intensity of grief. A score above 91 indicates severe grief (17). This measurement instrument has been widely used and validated around the world for many types of pregnancy loss, and has also been translated into several languages. Arabic, Chinese, French, German, Greek, Japanese, Portuguese, Spanish...

3 Statistical analysis :

The data were entered and analysed using Statistical Package for Social Science (SPSS) version 20 software. The normality of the data distribution was assessed using the Kolmogorov-Smirnov test. Continuous/quantitative variables were expressed as mean and standard deviation. On the other hand, categorical/qualitative variables were expressed in terms of numbers and frequencies. Differences between categorical variables were compared using Pearson's $\chi 2$ test or Fisher's exact test, as appropriate. The Mann-Whitney U test was used to compare differences between two independent groups when the independent variable was not normally distributed. The Kruskal-Wallis test was used. for comparisons involving more than two independent groups. The significance level was 5%.

4 Ethical considerations :

Before collecting any data, we obtained written authorisation from the head of the maternity department at CHU Hedi Chaker Sfax (see appendix 4). The students met with the woman and asked for her participation. The students explained to the woman the purpose of the study, the participation expected, their right not to answer certain questions, their right to withdraw from the study at any time or their right to refuse to participate. The questionnaire was also anonymous and confidential in order to ensure that the women could complete it properly.Data confidentiality was ensured throughout the study, as no names appeared on the questionnaires and a numerical code was used.

CHAPTER 3
RESULTS

A total of 109 women took part in this research. This section describes the socio-demographic characteristics of the respondents.

I. Descriptive section :

1 Socio-demographic characteristics :

1.1 Maternal age :

As Figure 1 shows, eight respondents are aged between 18 and 24, 41 women are over 35, while over half (n=60) are aged between 25 and 35. The average age of the women in our population is 32, with extremes of 18 and 58.

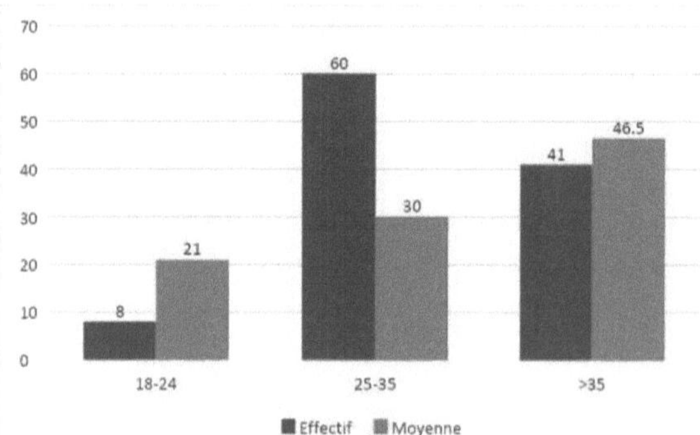

Figure 1: Age of the population

1.2 Origin :

In our study, we found that 63.9% (n=70) of the women were of urban origin (Figure 2).

8

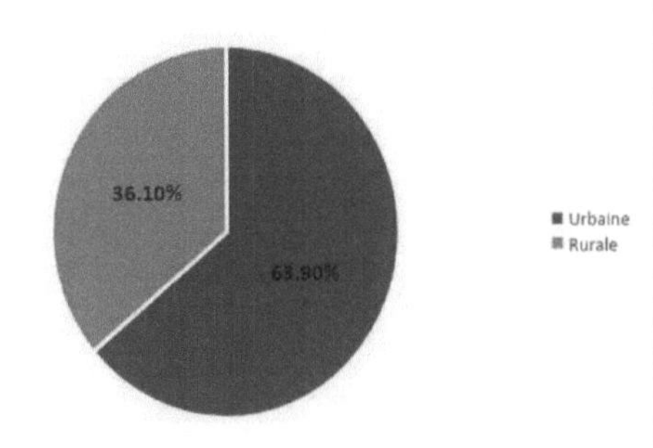

Figure 2: Origin of participants

1.3 Marital status :

In our population, 98.2% of women (n=107) were married. (Figure 3).

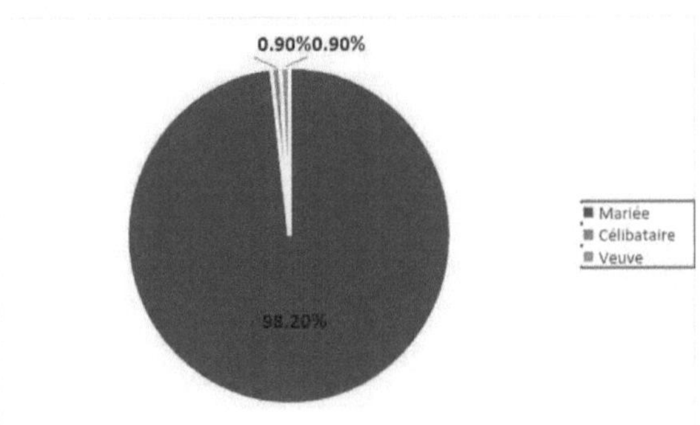

Figure 3: Marital status of women surveyed

1.4 Level of education :

With regard to level of education, 40.4% (n=44) had secondary education, 35.8% (n=39) had higher education, 19.3% (n=21) had primary education, and 4.6% (n=5) had never attended school, as shown in (Figure 4).

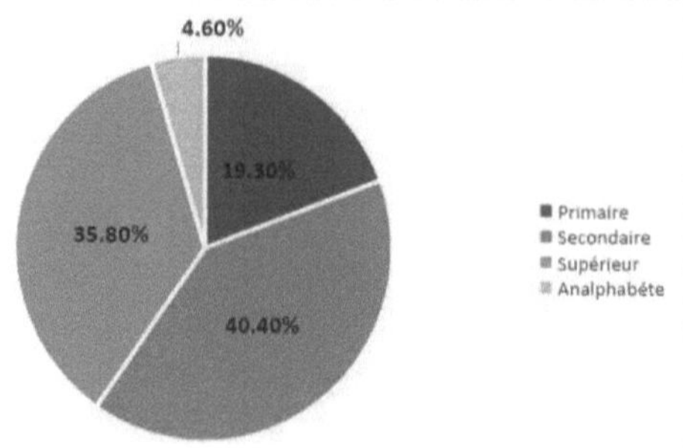

Figure 4: Level of education of participants

1.5 Women's occupations :

In our survey, the majority of women, 77.1% (n=84), were housewives (Figure 5).

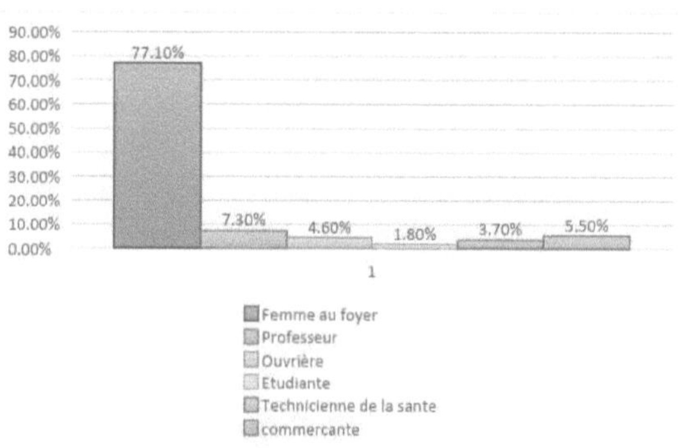

Figure 5: Occupation of women surveyed

1.6 Socio-economic level :

Eighty-three point five per cent of respondents (n=91) have an average socio-economic level. (Figure 7)

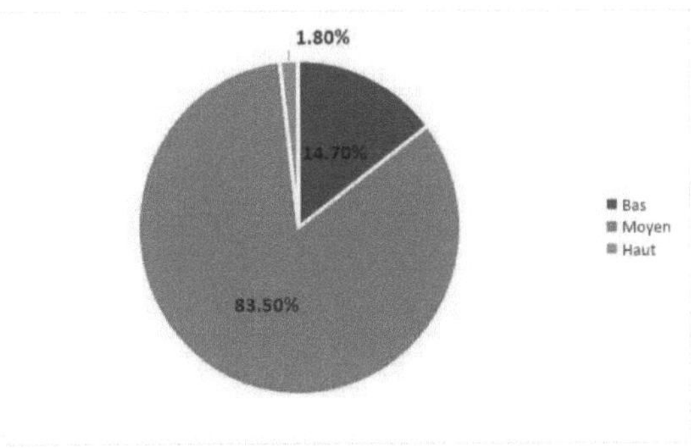

Figure 6: Socio-economic level of participants

2 Health and lifestyle/ Lifestyle :

2.1 BMI :

Almost half of the women (44%, n=48) had a BMI between 25 and 30, while 37.6% had a BMI between 18 and 25 (n=41) (Table 2).

Table 1: Distribution of patients according to BMI

BMI by interval	Number of employees (n)	Percentage (%)
Normal weight: [18, 5 - 25[.	41	37,6
Overweight: [25 - 30[.	47	43,1
Obesity: >=30	20	18, 3

2.2 Smoking :

Almost all the women surveyed, 97.20% (n=105), had never smoked (Figure 7).

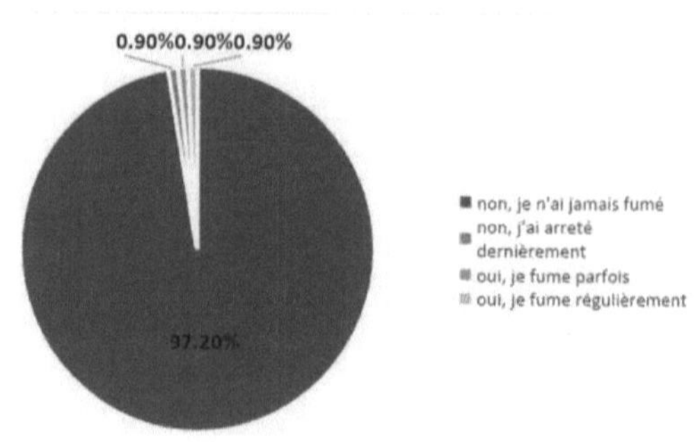

Figure 7: Percentage of women who smoke

2.3 Alcohol :

Almost all of our population, 99.1% (n=108), do not drink alcohol (Figure 8).

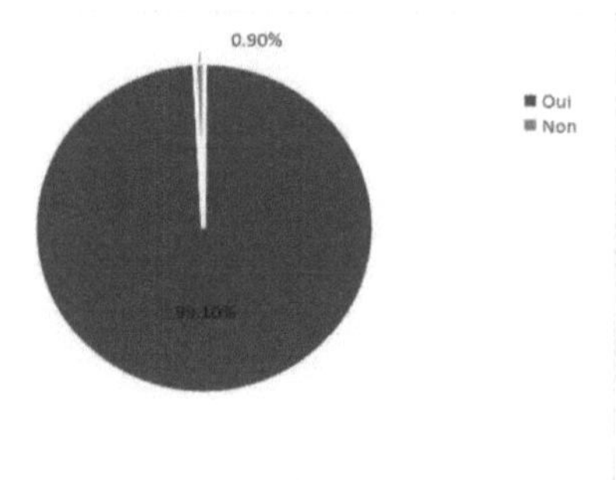

Figure 8: Notion of alcoholism in the study population

2.4 Medical history of the study population :

In our study, out of a total of 109 women, 79% (i.e. 86 women) had no disease, 5% were diabetic (n=5), 6% had thyroid disease (n=6), and 6% were hypertensive (n=7). (Figure 9)

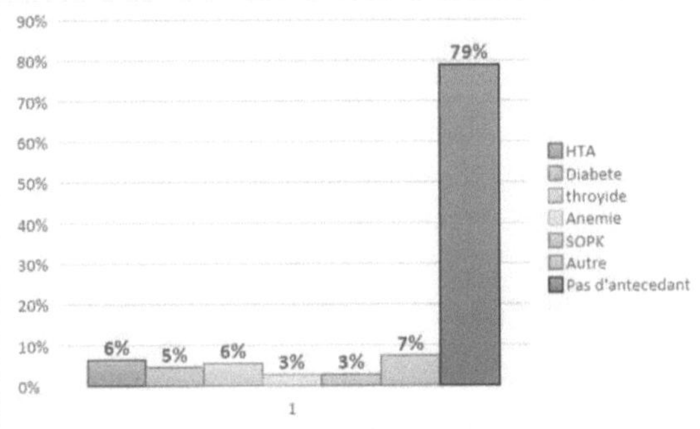

Figure 9: Medical history of women surveyed

2.5 Surgical history of the study population :

Most of the women (42.20%) had no previous surgical history, whereas 39.40% had undergone caesarean sections (Figure 10).

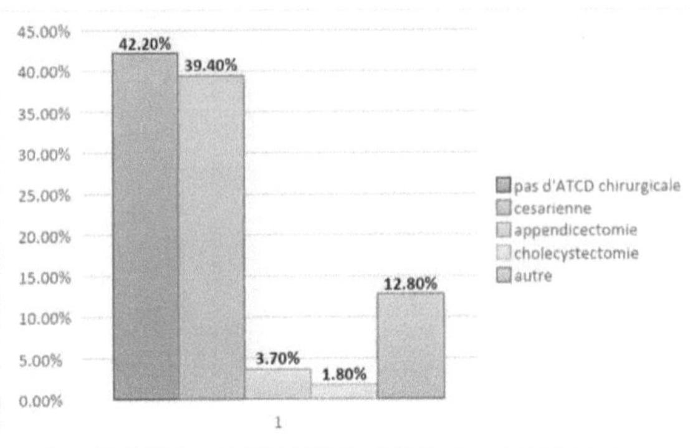

Figure 10: Surgical history of women surveyed

2.6 Gyneco-obstetrical history of the population studied

2.6.1 Gestité

More than half of the women surveyed were multi-gesture users, i.e. 66.1% (n=72). (Figure 11).

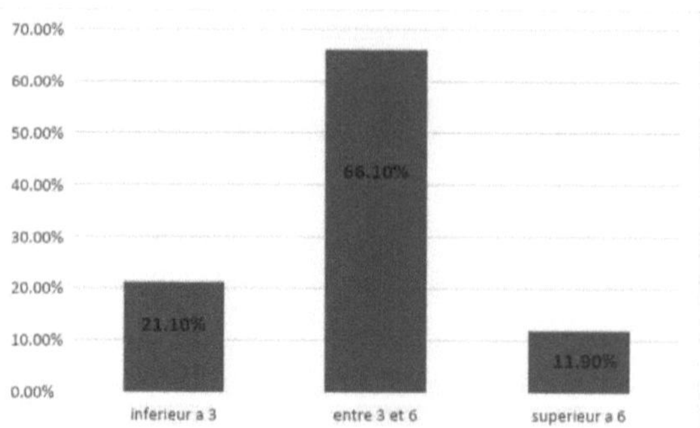

Figure 11: Breakdown of women by gender

2.6.2 Parity :

In this series, nulliparous women represented 7.3%, primiparous women 31.2%, multiparous women 57.8% and large multiparous women (parity > 4) only 3.7% (Figure12).

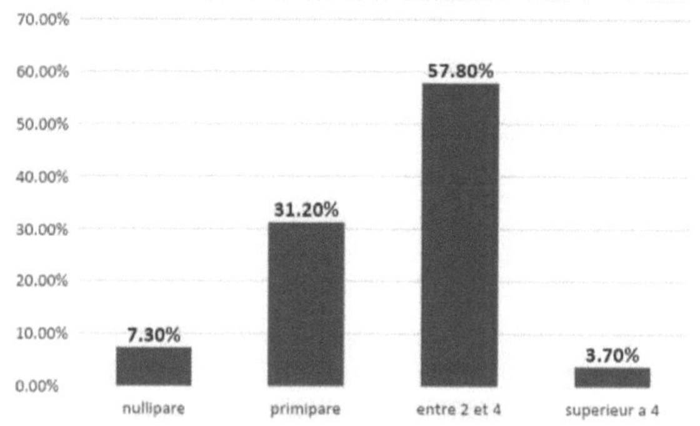

Figure 12: Breakdown of women by parity

2.6.3 Number of living children :

More than half the women (55%, n=60) have between 2 and 4 living children, 28.4% (n=31) have only one living child, 0.9% (n=1) have more than 4 and 15.6% (n=17) have no living children (Figure13).

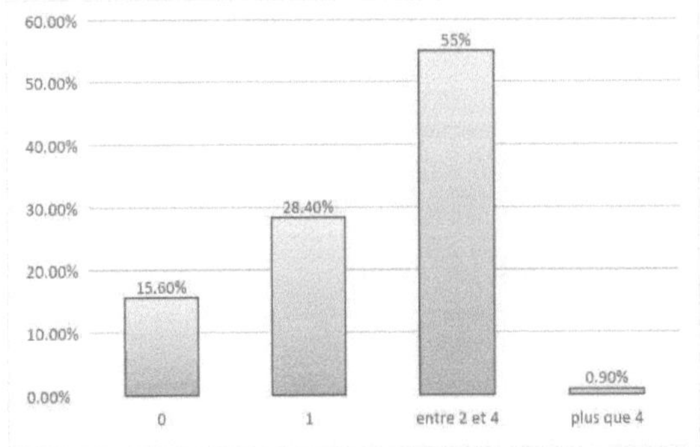

Figure 13: Breakdown of women by number of living children

2.6.4 Number of children who died :

8% (n=9) of women had only one child who died. (Figure 14)

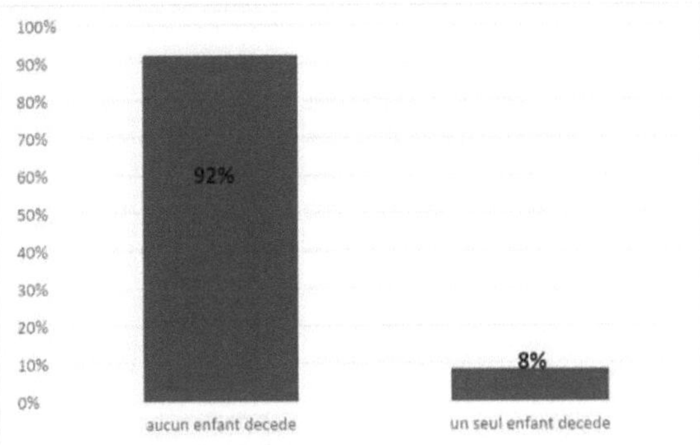

Figure 14: Breakdown of women by number of children who died

2.6.5 Delivery method :

Forty-seven point three per cent of women gave birth vaginally, while 52.7% delivered by caesarean section (Figure 15).

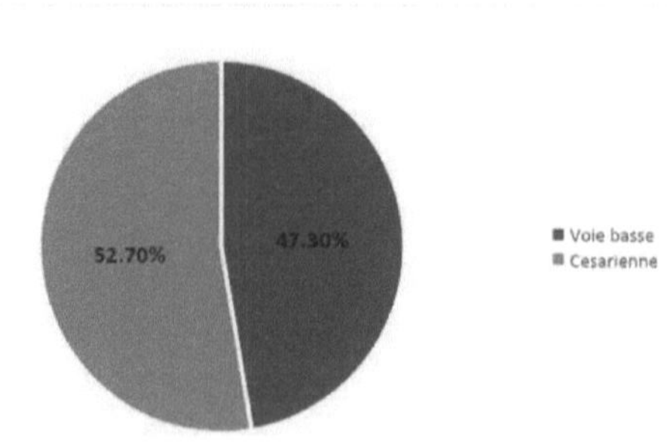

Figure 15: Mode of delivery

2.6.6 Number of caesarean sections :

Of those who underwent caesarean section (n =57): 19.3% (n =11) had a uni-cicatricial uterus and 26.6% (n =15) had a bi- to quadri-cicatricial uterus. (Figure 16)

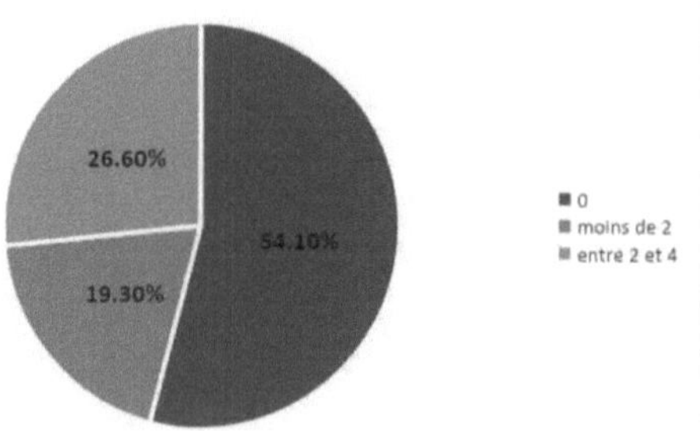

Figure 16: Number of caesarean sections

2.6.7 Concept of infertility :

Twenty-six point six per cent of women had a history of infertility. (Figure 17)

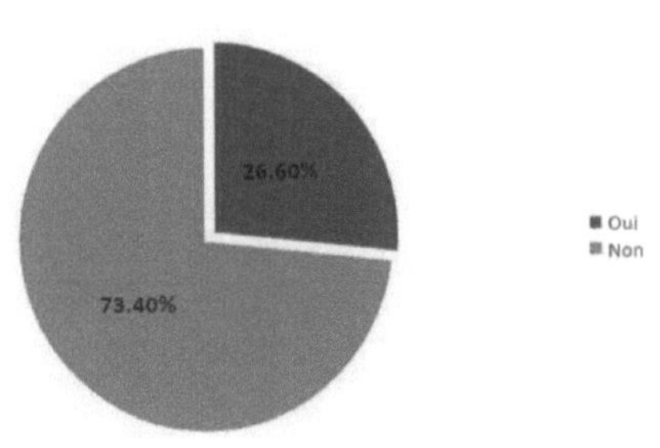

Figure 17: Concept of infertility

3 Information on miscarriages :

2.2   Number of miscarriages :

More than half the women had had a single miscarriage (56%), 33.9% had had two miscarriages and 9.2% had had more than three (Figure 18).

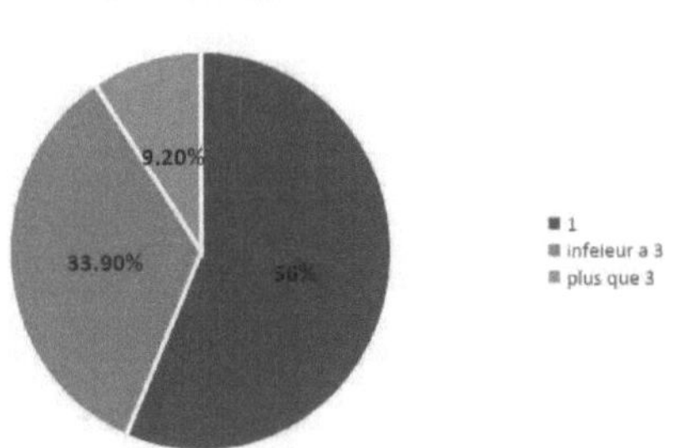

Figure 18: Number of miscarriages

3.2 Type of pregnancy lost: induced or spontaneous :

The majority of pregnancies were spontaneous (94.5%), while 5.5% (n=7) were induced (Figure 19).

- 4.6% by ovulation induction

- 0.9% by ICSI

- 0.9% by IVF

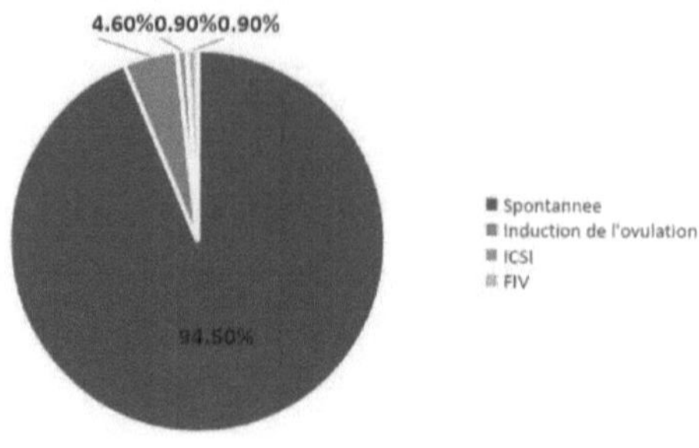

Figure 19: Type of pregnancy lost: induced or spontaneous

3.3 Stage of miscarriage

Table 2: Stage of miscarriage

	Before 12 weeks: complete and spontaneous	Before 12 weeks with curettage	After 12 weeks: complete and spontaneous	After 12 weeks with curettage	Total
1era FC	63,3%	21,1%	9,2 %	6,4 %	109 /109
2th FC	51,1%	19,1%	19,1%	10,6%	n= 47
3th FC	68,4%	10,5%	5,3%	15,8%	n= 19
4th FC	66,7%	16,7%	16,7%	-	n= 6
5th FC	33,3%	33,3%	33, 3%	-	n= 3
6th FC	-	-	-	-	n=1
7th FC	-	-	-	-	n=1
8th FC	-	-	-	-	n=1

3.4 Follow-up:

Almost all women (95.40%) (n=104) were followed up by a gynaecologist (Figure).

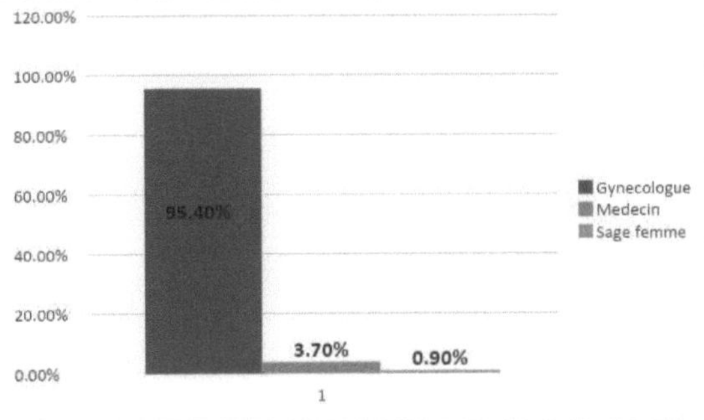

Figure 20: Breakdown of women by pregnancy follow-up provider

4 Support from professionals :

The majority of women (66 women, or 60.6% of the population) felt fully supported by healthcare professionals during the miscarriage(s) they had experienced. Six women said they were not supported at all (Figure 21).

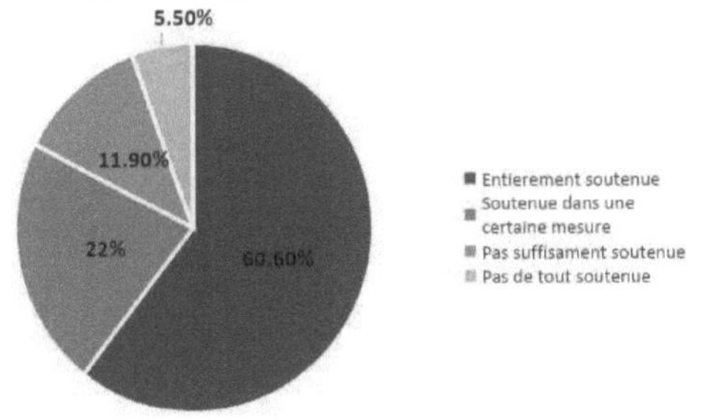

Figure 21: Support perceived by women from healthcare professionals during miscarriage(s)

5 Psychological support received from others :

In our population, the majority of women, 77.10% (n=84), received psychological support other than from healthcare professionals (Figure 22).

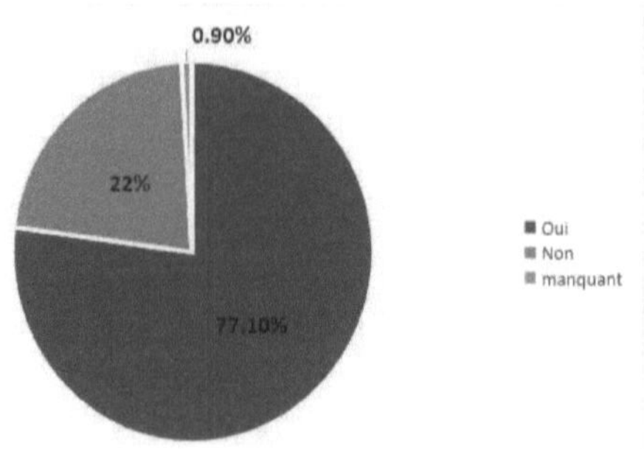

Figure 22: Breakdown of women who received psychological support in addition to that provided by a healthcare professional

This support was provided by the husband in 72% of cases (n=78), by family in 51% of cases (n=56), and by friends in 14% of cases (n=15) (Figure 23).

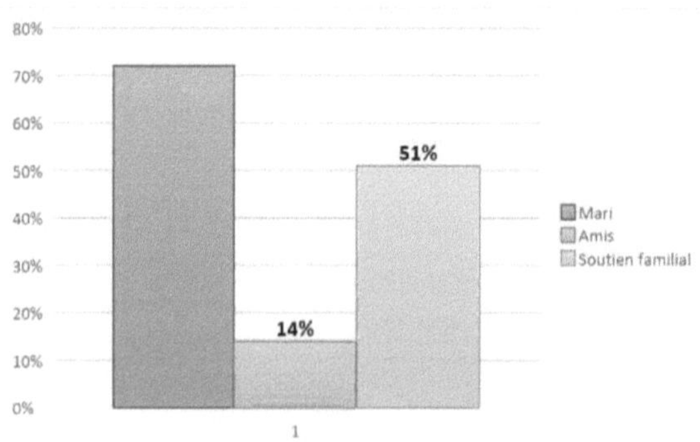

Figure 23: Breakdown of women by psychological support received from another person

6 Women's perceptions of the hospital following the management of their miscarriage :

35.8% of women had a negative perception of the hospital (Figure 24).

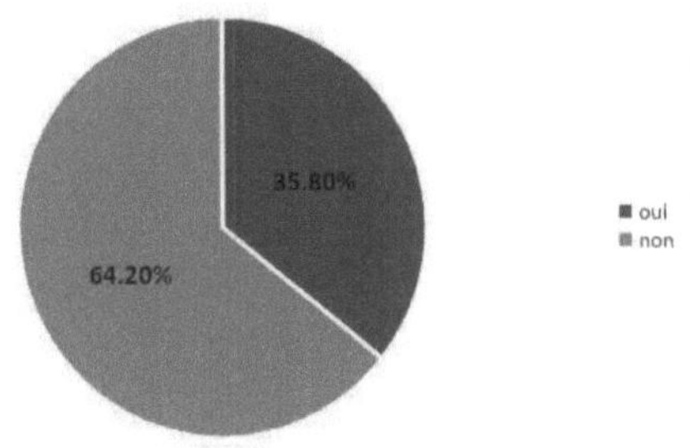

Figure 24: Women's perceptions of the hospital following the management of their miscarriage

These feelings lasted less than 3 months for 66.7% of women, between 3 and 6 months for 13.9% of them and more than 6 months for 19.4% of women (Figure 25).

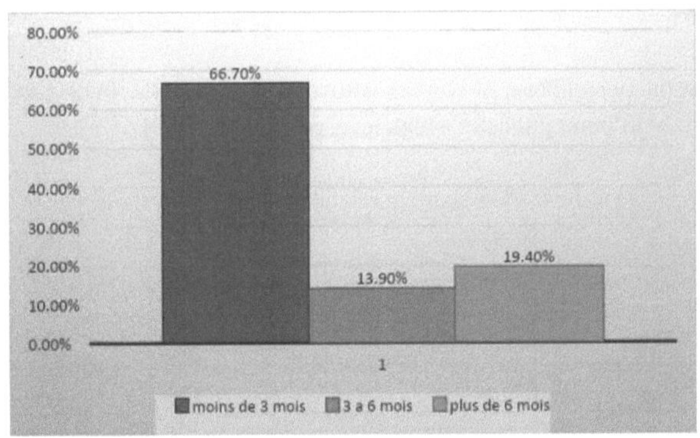

Figure 25: Duration of feelings

7 Psychological impact :

7.1 Perinatal bereavement: Perinatal bereavement scale :

The results observed among the 109 women on the Perinatal Bereavement Scale are presented in Table 7. Descriptive statistics, i.e. the minimum and maximum values of the scores obtained, as well as the mean and standard deviation, were calculated to describe the three dimensions of this scale. To better understand the values presented, it should be noted that the higher the values, the greater the perception of grief. The overall mean obtained was 103.57, with a significant standard deviation of 27.17, indicating a high degree of variation. The analysis reveals a level of "Acute grief" with a mean of 42.58 and a standard deviation of

11.58. However, for the "Coping" and "Hopelessness" dimensions, the scores were 42.15 and 30.43 respectively, with a lower mean than the "Acute grief" dimension. (Table 8)

Table 3: Women's scores on the perinatal bereavement scale

Dimensions of mourning	Average (SD)	Minimum	Maximum
Acute bereavement	42,15 (11,58)	14	55
Adaptation	30,43 (7,25)	16	46
Despair	31,06 (10,85)	11	51
Total bereavement scale perinatal	103,57 (27,17)	45	152

PGS = Perinatal Grief Scale SD: standard deviation

Severe PGS score

It was found that the percentages of women with total scores on the PGS ≥ 91 was 67.9%. A score above this cut-off point indicates a high level of grief (Table 9).

Table 4: PGS score in relation to the 91 threshold

	Workforce	Percentage
Score < 91 Score ≥ 91	35	32,1%
	74	67,9 %
Total	109	100

7.2 Concentration :

Forty-five point nine per cent of the women found it occasionally difficult to collect their thoughts and 33.9% had no difficulty concentrating (Table 6).

Table 5: Disruption to concentration experienced by women

	Workforce	Percentage (%)
No concentration difficulties	37	33,9
Occasional difficulty gathering thoughts	50	45,9
Difficulty concentrating and thinking straight	22	20,2

8 Physical impact :

8.1 Sleep :

More than half of the women (58.7%) reported slight difficulty in falling asleep after the miscarriage (Table 5).

Table 6: Sleep disturbance experienced

	Workforce	Percentage (%)
Sleeping as usual	33	30,3
Slight difficulty in falling asleep or reduced sleep	64	58,7
Reduced or interrupted sleep for at least 2 hours	11	10,1
Less than two or three hours' sleep	1	0,9

8.2 Appetite :

Sixty-three point three per cent of women reported a slightly reduced appetite following the miscarriage(s) (Table 7).

Table 7: Changes in appetite experienced by women

	Workforce	Percentage (%)
Normal or increased appetite	35	32,1
Slightly reduced appetite	69	63,3
No appetite, bland food	3	2,8
Need encouragement to eat	2	1,8

8.3 Post-abortive infertility:

Twenty-three point nine per cent of women (26 women) had consulted a doctor for post-abortive infertility (Figure 27).

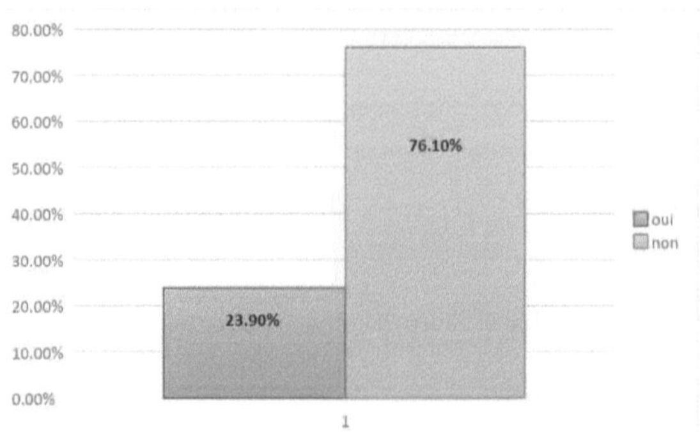

Figure 26: Women consulted for post-abortive infertility

8.4   Vaginismus :

Forty-four per cent of women reported that they had experienced post-abortive vaginismus (Figure 26).

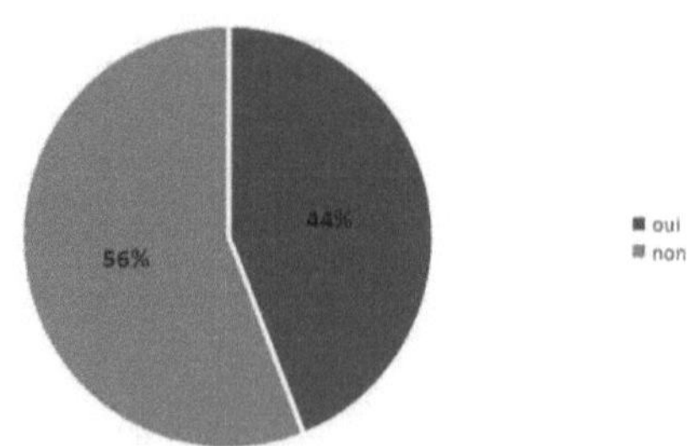

Figure 27: Breakdown of women reporting post-abortive vaginismus

8.5 Other complications:

Pelvic pain was the most common complication after miscarriage, reported by 51% of women. 34% of women had no complications (Figure28).

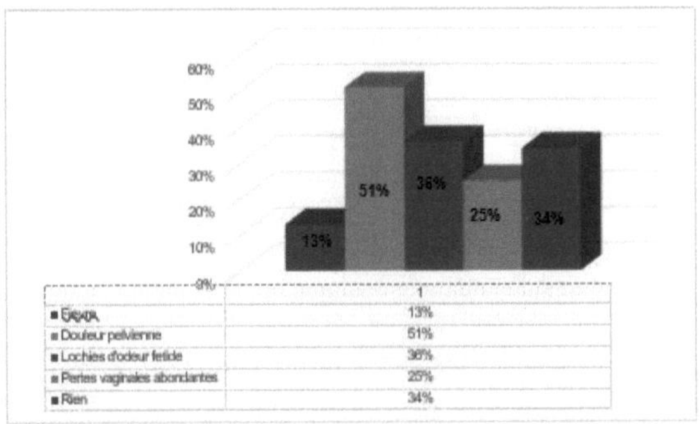

Figure 28: Physical complications reported by women following miscarriage(s)

9 The consequences of miscarriage for married life :

9.1 Husband's reaction:

Analysis of the results shows that the majority of spouses were supportive and understanding (80%), while 12% adopted a passive, withdrawn attitude towards their wife's experiences (Table 4).

Table 8: Husbands' reactions to their wives' experiences

Husband's reaction	Workforce	Percentage (%)
Emotionally affected and sad	59	54
Expressing feelings of guilt	3	3
Supportive and understanding	87	80
Passive and withdrawn	13	12

9.2 The impact of miscarriage on a woman's relationship with her partner :

In the majority of cases, i.e. 78.9%, the women stated that there had been no change in their relationship with their partners. However, 6.4% of women reported that their marital relationship had deteriorated after the miscarriage (Figure 29).

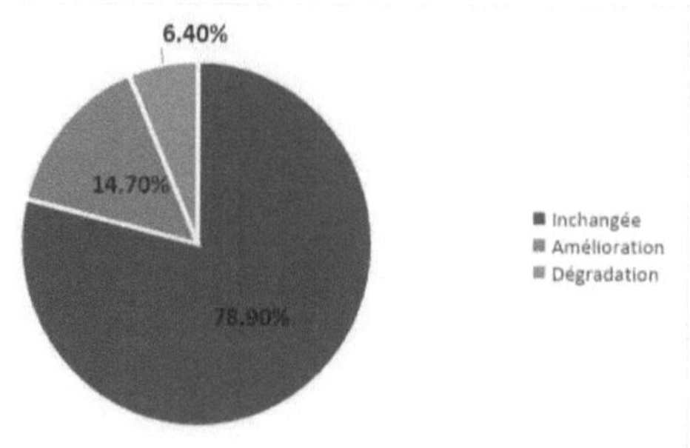

Figure 29: Impact of miscarriage on a woman's relationship with her partner

9.3 Impact of miscarriage on a woman's sex life :

In addition, intimate relations were influenced by this event. Six women reported that they had refused sex since their miscarriage (Figure 30).

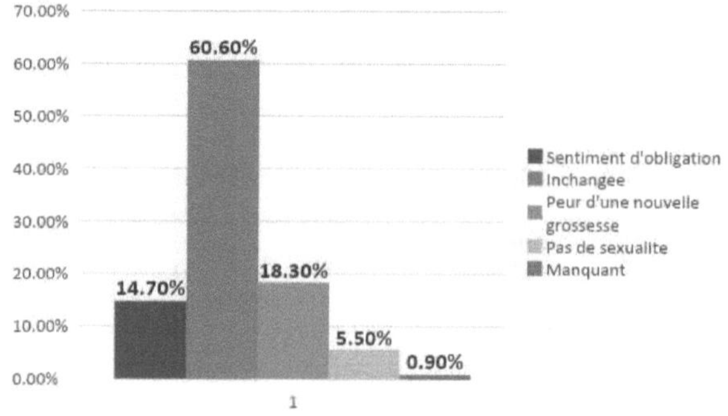

Figure 30: Impact of miscarriage on a woman's sex life

II. Analytical part :

1 The distribution of the total PGS score as a function of certain socio-demographic variables :

A statistically significant difference was found between the mean values of the PGS total score in terms of the "origin" variable (P= 0.029 < 0.05).

Table 9: Distribution of the total PGS score according to certain socio-demographic variables

		N	Average	Standard deviation	Test	Statistical significance Value of P
	Age					
Score of PGS	18 - 24	8	121,25	14,01	χ2= 2,19	0,334
	25 - 34	60	101,23	28,51		
	>=35	41	103,53	26,26		
	Origin Urban	69	99,22	27,05	Z= -2,188	0,029*
	Rural	39	110,64	26,22		
	Professional status No	84	101,49	27,88	Z=-1,405	0,160
	Yes	25	110,56	26,85		

PGS = Perinatal Grief Scale ;

* : significant p < 0.05 ;

Z = Mann-Whitney U test; χ2= Kruskal Wallis test ;

2 The distribution of the total PGS score as a function of certain medical and obstetric variables :

The table below shows that a statistically significant difference was found between the mean values of the total scores on the PGS in terms of the number of miscarriages (P = 0.020 =< 0.05).

Table 10: Distribution of the total PGS score as a function of certain medical and obstetric variables

		N	Average	Standard deviation	Test	Statistical significance Value of P
GSP score	ATCD MP Yes No	23 86	103,09 103,70	31,33 26,15	Z= -,048	0,961
	Fertility problems Yes No	29 80	107,38 102,19	26,32 27,51	Z= -,960	0,337
	Living child Yes	17	103,14	27,60	Z= -,413	0,679
	No	92	105,88	25,36		
	Number of CF1[2-3] >3	61 37 10	96,74 112,97 111,20	28,40 23,54 22,70	χ2= 7,82	0,020*
	Type of pregnancy lost Spontaneous Induced	103 6	103,37 106,83	27,09 31,07	Z= -,292	0,770

PGS = Perinatal Grief Scale ;

* : significant p < 0.05 ;

Z = Mann-Whitney U test; χ2= Kruskal Wallis test; PD = personal medical history

Table 12 shows the mean perinatal bereavement scores as a function of time since miscarriage. The non-parametric Kruskal-Wallis test revealed no significant difference in mean scores according to time since miscarriage ($\chi2= 0.48$), p = .922).

Table 11: Time since miscarriage

	Time since miscarriage				Chi-square 2	ddl	p
	0-6 months	7-12 months	1-2 years	>2 years			
Bereavement score perinatal	107,67	105,21	103,29	102,61	0,48	3	0,922

χ2= Kruskal Wallis test

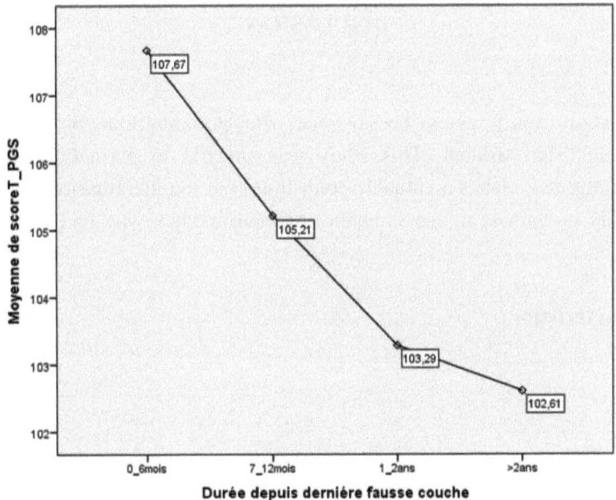

Figure 31: Changes in average perinatal bereavement scores as a function of time since miscarriage

CHAPTER 4
DISCUSSION

The aim of this study was to assess bereavement after perinatal loss, more specifically after miscarriage, in Tunisian women. This study was specific to perinatal bereavement in a retrospective manner and makes a valuable contribution to the literature on bereavement, as it was the first study in Tunisia to assess bereavement in women who had experienced one or more miscarriages.

1 Patient characteristics :

1.1 Age :

We interviewed 109 women of Tunisian nationality, all of whom were included in this analysis. At the time of the interview, participants were aged between 18 and 58 years. In this study, the highest prevalence of miscarriage was among women aged 25 to 35 (55%). The prevalence of miscarriage was lowest among women aged 18 to 24 (7.3%).These figures are partly consistent with a study conducted in Saudi Arabia, which aimed to estimate the prevalence and maternal age, as well as other risk factors for miscarriage among Sudanese women. The results of this study showed that the highest prevalence of miscarriage was among women aged between 25 and 34 (58.6%). The lowest prevalence was among women under 20 (2.4%) (20). Moreover, it has been established that advanced maternal age is a major risk factor for miscarriage: the risk of miscarriage increases from the age of 30, reaching 53% when the woman's age is 45 or over(21). However, our study did not specifically examine women over 35 separately, but the high prevalence among women aged 25 to 35 is in line with trends observed elsewhere.

2 Health and lifestyle :

2.1 BMI :

Body mass index (BMI) is calculated by dividing weight in kilograms by the square of height in metres. The BMI categories used in this The analysis is as follows: 18.5 to 24.9 (normal weight), 25.0 to 29.9 (overweight) and 30.0 or more (obese) (22). These categories are defined by the World Health Organisation and the US National Institute of Health(23) . Obesity has a major impact on female fertility, and this has been demonstrated in the literature. Indeed, there is an observed difference in pregnancy loss between obese women and the general population. (Boots & Stephenson, 2011) (Metwally et al., 2010) (24). The results of this study indicate that the majority (43.1%) of women who experienced a miscarriage were overweight, with a BMI between 25 and 30. The risk of miscarriage among women with a higher BMI (overweight) in this study is in line with previous studies conducted in Nepal in 2020 (25), in London (26), at Sheffield Hospital in the UK (27) and in the north of England (30).

30

2.2 Alcohol and tobacco :

In this study, all our women were neither alcoholics nor smokers, which may be explained by socio-cultural and religious factors. A study conducted in Denmark in 2023 showed no association between excessive alcohol consumption and the risk of miscarriage in either the first or second trimester (28). However, research carried out in the state of Tennessee (United States) in 2019 revealed an association between exposure to alcohol and a dose-dependent increase in the risk of miscarriage. In addition, a systematic review highlighted that excessive alcohol consumption during the first trimester of pregnancy is linked to a higher likelihood of miscarriage (29). With regard to smoking, a previous study showed that the risk of miscarriage in women aged 25-29 years was not associated with exposure to tobacco smoke, whereas all other age groups showed an increased risk in the presence of active smoking (30). However, other research confirms that smoking is an important modifiable risk factor for miscarriage, with an increased risk especially when it occurs during pregnancy. This risk increases with the amount of tobacco consumed, with an increase in relative risk of 1% for each cigarette smoked per day {Citation}.

2.3 Signs that led the woman to consult :

Our results show that women have bodily sensations that are suggestive of an early miscarriage. The main signs are bleeding (81%), which can be light (31%) or heavy (50%), and pelvic pain. This study is in agreement with another study carried out in France in 2014 by Camille (31), which shows that the three main signs suggestive of miscarriage are bleeding, pelvic pain and diminishing signs of pregnancy. However, it is not necessarily the presence of these signs that leads women to seek medical advice (28%). This is in line with other studies, such as those by Limbo, Glasser and Sundaram (2014), which have shown that it is women's intuition that alerts them to possible signs of miscarriage (32).

3 Use of psychological support :

The results show that a significant number of women (77.1%) seek psychological support from those around them (family, friends). In this context, another study by Séjourné et al. showed that it is important for women to have their experiences validated by those around them in order to resolve and integrate the loss (31). On the other hand, the study by Camille qu'showed that the people around them are not always aware of the loss, because women find it difficult to deal with their reactions, which are mostly indifferent and awkward. This difference can be explained by cultural variations. In some cultures, from the day of the wedding, the whole entourage awaits the arrival of the "crown prince" (31).

4 Bad impression of the hospital:

Analysis of the results shows that some parents noted a lack of empathy and a minimisation, even a lack of recognition, of their loss by healthcare professionals in the emergency services, which gave them the impression that their situation was not taken seriously (35.8%). (33)In this context, a Canadian study carried out in 2021 by Emond Tina showed that professional attitudes and behaviour and the comments and behaviour of healthcare professionals contribute to the negative emotions felt by parents.

5 Psychological repercussions of miscarriage

5.1 Perinatal bereavement: The perinatal bereavement scale

An important aspect of the PGS is its ability to differentiate between women who are going through a typical bereavement process and those who may be prone to more severe consequences following their loss. A normal bereavement process will be characterised by lower acute grief scores and higher coping and hopelessness s c o r e s (34). In the present study, we found a higher mean acute grief score than mean hopelessness and mean adjustment scores, with a mean total score of 103.57, indicating that our participants had a severe grief process. These results are in contradiction with another Thai study, which found mean acute grief scores were lower compared to mean coping and mean hopelessness scores (35).

5.2 High perinatal bereavement (PGS) ≥ 91 :

The study population comprised 109 women, more than half (67.9%) of whom were experiencing high grief at the time of the interview, with a score greater than or equal to the cut-off point of 91. A study of women with pregnancy loss in Turkey, regardless of the duration of pregnancy, found that 55.7% of women with pregnancy loss had perinatal grief scores (PGS) ≥ 91 immediately after the loss (T0). This percentage decreased to 21.1% at the third month (T1), 3.5% at the sixth month (T2) and remained at 3.5% one year after discharge (T3) (36).

5.3 Concentration :

Analysis of our results showed that early miscarriage has psychological repercussions. A significant number of women (66.1%) reported concentration difficulties of varying intensity after the miscarriage. Our results are in line with data collected in other studies, which have clearly shown that perinatal bereavement also puts parents at risk of developing psychological or somatic problems, such as partial denial of reality, inability to concentrate and memory problems (37).

6 Physical consequences of miscarriage :

Analysis of the data shows that early miscarriage can lead to a number of physical disturbances.

6.1 Sleep and appetite :

In terms of sleep disturbance, 69.7% of bereaved women suffered from sleep disturbance (difficulty falling asleep and/or reduced sleep). In addition, 63.3% of women reported a reduction in appetite. These are the physical impacts of this type of bereavement. Physical consequences such as sleep disturbances, lack of appetite, fatigue, feelings of suffocation and chest pain have been widely documented in the scientific literature and have been observed in some parents after the loss of a child(38) (39).These results are also in line with another more recent qualitative study conducted in Quebec by Aissatou Djiba, which showed that the respondents experienced numerous difficulties affecting various dimensions of their physical and psychological health during the various stages of the grieving process. On the physical level, some respondents experienced difficulties such as chronic fatigue and sleep disorders (40).

6.2 Post-abortive infertility:

Post-abortive infertility is generally seen in women who were already infertile before the miscarriage.Of the 26.6% of women in our study followed for infertility, 23.9% consulted for post-abortive infertility. These results are in line with another study carried out in Athens by Anastasia Tzonou et al, which showed that women who had developed secondary infertility were already sub-fertile and had a higher frequency of miscarriage (41).

6.3 Vaginismus :

This study reveals that a significant number of bereaved women reported having developed post-abortive vaginismus (44%). This can be explained in part by feelings of fear related to another pregnancy or miscarriage. One possible explanation for the association between vaginismus and the psychological disturbances experienced by the women in our population is that vaginismus may be a physical manifestation of the emotional distress experienced during perinatal bereavement. Bereaved women may experience great anxiety, fear and feelings of helplessness after a miscarriage, which may contribute to the development of vaginismus. Vaginismus may be the body's protective reaction to these negative emotions, where the vaginal muscles involuntarily contract in response to fear or anxiety, making sexual intercourse painful or even impossible. Thus, high grief and associated psychological disorders can create a vicious circle where vaginismus worsens emotional distress, which in turn can reinforce vaginismus. However, the literature on this subject is poor, and there is great interest in exploring this association further.

7 The consequences of miscarriage for married life

7.1 Relationship with husband :

Analysis of the data shows that miscarriages can have a variable impact on couples, with 21.1% of women reporting a deterioration in their relationship with their partner since the event. In fact, the difference in the intensity of mothers' and fathers' grief reactions can sometimes have significant repercussions on the family life and couple relationships of bereaved parents (42) (Lang et al., 2011; Lang et al., 1996; Mekosh-Rosenbaum & Lasker, 1995; Zeanah et al., 1995). A study of 185 women during the first year following a perinatal loss revealed that 32% of them noted a deterioration in their interpersonal relationships and 39% recognised difficulties related to their marital intimacy (Swanson et al., 2003) (40).

However, some of the women in this study felt that despite this difficult event, their relationship with their partner had improved and reported that their husbands had become more tender, understanding and supportive (14.7%). This finding is consistent with another study by Francine De Montigny, et al, which showed that a significant number of women reported that their relationship had become closer and more supportive after a perinatal loss. Several other researchers have also suggested that the many challenges faced by bereaved parents could, in some cases, have a positive influence on their relationship (40).

7.2 Sexuality:

With regard to the feeling or experience of intimate relations after the miscarriage, our study revealed that the majority of participants (60.6%) did not notice any change. However, some women reported a negative impact on their sexuality, manifested by a feeling of obligation (14.7%) and fear of another pregnancy (18.3%). Other studies have found that distance in interpersonal and sexual relationships was associated with greater emotional disturbance in women, including more depressed, anxious, confused and angry moods. As already suggested by Speraw (43) (44), Beutel et al (45) and others (46) (47). In addition, Séjourné and Call state that 51% of women experience anxiety about future pregnancies, as well as a negative impact on the couple and their sexuality (3).

Analytical part :

1. Perinatal bereavement as a function of age :

This study found no significant difference in the average PGS score according to age. Both younger and older women still obtained similar results. On the other hand, a study conducted in Turkey in 2022 revealed that the age variable had a significant effect on the median total GSP score after loss. The total SGP score of women aged between 20 and 29 was higher than that of other age groups. (36). Similarly, Robert et al. emphasised that maternal age is an important predictor of sadness, highlighting a negative relationship between maternal age and perinatal sadness(48).

2. Perinatal bereavement as a function of parity :

In our survey, we found that a significant number of women (57.8%) had a parity of between 2 and 4, which may be a risk factor for miscarriage. A recent study published in the journal BMC Pregnancy and Childbirth confirms that the number of miscarriages per woman increases with parity. In general, women with higher parities are also older than those with lower parities, which may explain this correlation (49). From the point of view of the association between psychological symptoms, perinatal bereavement and parity, it should be noted that the factors associated with perinatal bereavement were not studied in our analysis. Analysis of the data shows that previous child ownership seems to slightly reduce the intensity of grief in women who have experienced a miscarriage. However, the non-parametric Mann-Whitney test did not reveal any significant difference in mean PGS scores according to parity (Z = -0.413, p = 0.679). It is important to note that not having living children has been consistently associated with increased levels of depressive symptoms, anxiety and bereavement (6) (50) (51). Neugebauer et al. reported that increased parity seems to protect againstdepression (6). For major depressive disorder following miscarriage, the relative risk was reported to be considerably higher in women without children (RR = 5.0; 95% CI: 1.7 to 14.4) than in women with children (RR = 1.3; 95% CI: 0.5 to 3.5). (50). This observation is in line with other studies carried out in France, which have shown that the experience of this event is less traumatic as a function of parity and the absence of a history of miscarriage (31).

3. Changes in Perinatal Bereavement Scores over time After a miscarriage :

In our study, we examined mean perinatal bereavement scores as a function of time since miscarriage. The results showed that the mean total score was 107.67 for women within 0 to 6 months of the miscarriage, then fell slightly to 105.21 for those between 7 and 12 months, to 103.29 for those between 1 and 2 years, and finally to 102.61 for those more than 2 years after the miscarriage. However, the Kruskal-Wallis test revealed no significant difference in mean scores according to the time elapsed since the miscarriage ($\chi2$= 0.48, p = 0.922). These results suggest that although the mean score decreases slightly over time, this decrease is not statistically significant. Levels of grief in women who have experienced pregnancy loss have been reported in the literature (52) (53) (54) (5) (55). And we found that our results were not in agreement with those found by the majority of studies which have shown that women experience different levels of grief immediately after a perinatal loss, and that this grief tends to diminish progressively over time(52) (54) (5) (56). In a qualitative study, Avelin et al. reported that after the loss of a baby, couples said they were still crying and in physical pain in the third month after the loss. One year later, however, they felt stronger(57). In contrast to these results, in our study we found that the women had a mean score of 105.21 even one year after the loss and 103.29 two years later, indicating that grief persisted over a longer period for some women.

STRENGTHS AND LIMITATIONS OF THE STUDY

In this chapter, the results obtained are examined in more detail and discussed in the context of the scientific literature. This chapter also discusses the strengths and limitations of the study. Finally, recommendations for clinical practice, training and research and a conclusion are discussed in the last section.

1 Study strengths :

Our study includes a sample of 109 women, which provides a solid basis for robust statistical analysis and allows potential generalisations to a wider population. This sample size reduces bias and strengthens the reliability of the conclusions. In addition, the consistency of some of our results with those of the existing literature reinforces the validity of our observations and their relevance in the wider context of research into miscarriage and its impacts.Our study is the first to assess levels of bereavement among women who have experienced miscarriage in Tunisia, while describing the psychological, physical and relational consequences of this event. This holistic approach highlights the overall impact of miscarriage on Tunisian women, adding significant value to the existing literature and paving the way for future research.We used a Perinatal Bereavement Scale (PGS), validated and widely used in the literature on perinatal bereavement. The use of this tool increases the reliability of our results, enabling solid comparisons with other studies in this field.

2 Limitations of the study :

We included all women who had experienced a miscarriage, regardless of the length of time since the event. As a result, women may have difficulty recalling details of their miscarriage accurately, which could affect the reliability of the data collected by introducing recall bias. Participants may tend to give answers that they consider socially acceptable or expected rather than accurately describing their actual experience and feelings. This social desirability bias could distort the results by overestimating the positive impacts or minimising the negative ones. The sample was made up of women from the same health establishment (uni-centric study), so the results may not be generalizable to the entire Tunisian female population.As the study is based on cross-sectional data, it does not allow us to monitor changes in the psychological and physical impact of miscarriage over the long term. A longitudinal study would be necessary to observe these changes over time. We used a non-probability convenience sampling method. This method may introduce selection bias and limit the generalisation of results to a wider population.

RECOMMENDATIONS

The results of this study will enable us to make relevant recommendations f o r practice, research and training.

1 Recommendations for clinical practice :

1. Educate healthcare professionals, including gynaecologists, midwives and psychologists, about the psychological and physical consequences of miscarriage.
2. Make medical staff aware of the signs of bereavement and psychological distress in women who have suffered a miscarriage, so that they can provide appropriate support.
3. Train staff on the risk factors predisposing to psychological morbidity, such as a history of psychiatric illness, childlessness, lack of social support, poor marital adjustment, previous pregnancy loss and ambivalence towards the foetus.
4. Carers need to be aware of the possible moderating effect of clinical practices, such as surgical treatment and ultrasound findings, on the psychological impact of miscarriage.
5. The woman experiencing a miscarriage must be given adequate information about the cause (where such information exists) and the implications of the miscarriage for future chances of conception and successful delivery. Reassurance is also necessary. Women should be informed of the possible physical symptoms they may experience in the weeks following the miscarriage, as well as the potential psychological symptoms such as grief, depression and anxiety that may follow.
6. Include a systematic assessment of mental health in post-miscarriage care, using validated tools such as the Perinatal Grief Scale (PGS).
7. Offer psychological support and counselling services from the time of the miscarriage diagnosis and during post-miscarriage follow-up, to help women manage their grief and prevent long-term complications.
8. Encourage joint consultations where both partners can express their feelings and concerns. This helps to strengthen communication and mutual support.
9. Offering couple therapy sessions for couples experiencing difficulties in their relationship after a miscarriage, in order to prevent tension and improve the marital relationship.
10. Provide information on available community resources, such as helplines, support associations and online forums.
11. Develop educational brochures and workshops that explain the different stages of perinatal bereavement and offer strategies for coping with the emotional and relational challenges.

2 Recommendations for research :

Given the lack of specific studies on miscarriage in our country, and on the experiences and needs of women and their families in this context, we suggest the following directions for research:

➤ Carry out in-depth qualitative studies to explore the experiences of Tunisian women after a miscarriage, focusing on their needs, concerns and available resources.

➤ Carrying out longitudinal studies to monitor the evolution of perinatal bereavement in Tunisian women over time, examining the risk and protective factors associated with psychological adaptation.

➤ To examine the role of family members, including partners and relatives, in the bereavement process of women following a miscarriage. This will enable us to better understand family dynamics and develop family-centred interventions.

➤ Exploring fathers' experiences after miscarriage and their need for support. It is essential to include fathers' perspectives in research and to develop interventions that meet their specific needs.

➤ To evaluate the effectiveness of different forms of support, including individual support, educational programmes and online interventions, for women and families affected by miscarriage.

➤ Develop and evaluate interventions specifically adapted to the Tunisian cultural context, taking into account local beliefs, social norms and traditions.

3 Training recommendation :

In response to the shortcomings identified in the studies concerning the lack of knowledge and training of healthcare professionals in the management of women who have suffered a miscarriage, as well as the insufficient emphasis placed on emotional care, we propose the following recommendations for initial and continuing training.

Initial training :

• Integration of modules on miscarriage and perinatal bereavement:

Include modules dedicated to miscarriage, perinatal bereavement and the psychological impact of these events in initial training programmes for health professionals, particularly in medical, midwifery, psychology and counselling courses.

• Empathic communication training :

Offer specific training in empathic communication and the helping relationship to enable future healthcare professionals to interact sensitively and compassionately with women and families affected by miscarriage.

Continuing education :

• Workshops and seminars on the management of miscarriages:

Organising regular workshops and seminars for healthcare professionals to enhance their skills in the overall care of women who have experienced a miscarriage, with a particular focus on the emotional and relational aspects.

• Sharing best practice and recent research:

To facilitate the sharing of best practice and recent research in the field of miscarriage management through conferences, publications and online platforms dedicated to continuing education.

CONCLUSION

Miscarriage or spontaneous abortion is the most common complication of pregnancy, affecting one in four women (58). Even if the miscarriage occurs very early and the pregnancy was not yet visible, for many women it represents the loss of a future baby and of all the plans it had for the future. It is in this context that our study assessed the level of perinatal mourning and studied the physical and psychological consequences of miscarriage for Tunisian women.The loss of a pregnancy is a traumatic experience that can lead to deep and lasting grief, as indicated by the high perinatal bereavement scores and cognitive difficulties reported by women. Our results thus highlight the crucial importance of psychological care for women bereaved after a miscarriage. Healthcare professionals, including midwives, play a key role in supporting women who have experienced a miscarriage. They should be trained to recognise and assess signs of psychological distress in bereaved women, offer appropriate emotional support and refer patients to specialist mental health services if necessary. It is also essential to facilitate support groups and educational resources to help women navigate through their bereavement, as well as promoting open and empathetic communication, ensuring that women feel heard and supported during this difficult time. In conclusion, a holistic approach integrating psychological and physical care is essential to help women overcome the grief associated with a miscarriage. Healthcare professionals, and midwives in particular, are in the front line in providing this crucial support.

REFERENCES

1. bfs.admin.ch/bfs/en/home/statistics/catalogues-banks-data/definitions.assetdetail.5936332.htm [Internet]. [cited 22 May 2024]. Available from: https://www.bfs.admin.ch/bfs/fr/home/statistiques/catalogues-banques-%20data/definitions.assetdetail.5936332.htm

2. Methods of managing miscarriage: a network meta-analysis - Ghosh, J - 2021 | Cochrane Library [Internet]. [cited 22 May 2024]. Available from: https://www.cochranelibrary.com/cdsr/doi/10.1002/14651858.CD012602.pub2/full/fr

3. Séjourné N, Callahan S, Chabrol H. L'impact psychologique de la fausse couche : revue de travaux. Journal of Gynaecology Obstetrics and Reproductive Biology. 1 Sept 2008;37(5):435-40.

4. The Lancet - 2021 - Miscarriage worldwide reform of care is needed.pdf [Internet]. [cited 22 May 2024]. Available from: https://www.thelancet.com/pdfs/journals/lancet/PIIS0140-6736(21)00954-5.pdf

5. deMontigny F, Verdon C, Meunier S, Dubeau D. Women's persistent depressive and perinatal grief symptoms following a miscarriage: the role of childlessness and satisfaction with healthcare services. Arch Womens Ment Health. 2017;20(5):655-62.

6. Neugebauer R, Kline J, O'Connor P, Shrout P, Johnson J, Skodol A, et al. Determinants of depressive symptoms in the early weeks after miscarriage. Am J Public Health. Oct 1992;82(10):1332-9.

7. Romano H, Aurore A, Chollet-Xemard C, Marty J. Psychological issues of perinatal death in prehospital emergency medicine. Ann Fr Med Urgence. 1 March 2011;1(2):123-30.

8. Romano H, Aurore A, Chollet-Xémard C, Marty J. Psychological issues of perinatal death in prehospital emergency medicine. Annales françaises de médecine d'urgence. 1 March 2011;1:123-30.

9. Kersting A, Wagner B. Complicated grief after perinatal loss. Dialogues in Clinical Neuroscience. 30 June 2012;14(2):187-94.

10. Brier N. Grief Following Miscarriage: A Comprehensive Review of the Literature. Journal of Women's Health. Apr 2008;17(3):451-64.

11. Lok IH, Yip ASK, Lee DTS, Sahota D, Chung TKH. A 1-year longitudinal study of psychological morbidity after miscarriage. Fertil Steril. Apr 2010;93(6):1966-75.

12. Beutel M, Deckardt R, von Rad M, Weiner H. Grief and depression after miscarriage: their separation, antecedents, and course. Psychosom Med. 1995;57(6):517-26.

13. Previous prenatal loss as a predictor of perinatal depression and anxiety - PubMed

[Internet]. [cited 22 May 2024]. Available from: https://pubmed.ncbi.nlm.nih.gov/21372060/

14. BHUGRA D, BECKER MA. Migration, cultural bereavement and cultural identity. World Psychiatry. Feb 2005;4(1):18-24.

15. Hollins Martin C. Bereavement Care for Childbearing Women and their Families: An Interactive Workbook. Bereavement Care for Childbearing Women and their Families: An Interactive Workbook. 2013.

16. Murray JA, Terry DJ, Vance JC, Battistutta D, Connolly Y. Effects of a program of intervention on parental distress following infant death. Death Stud. June 2000;24(4):275-305.

17. Toedter LJ, Lasker JN, Alhadeff JM. The Perinatal Grief Scale: development and initial validation. Am J Orthopsychiatry. July 1988;58(3):435-49.

18. Toedter LJ, Lasker JN, Alhadeff JM. Perinatal Grief Scale [Internet]. 2011 [cited 22 May 2024]. Available from: https://doi.apa.org/doi/10.1037/t04871-000

19. Perinatal Grief Scale, Scoring and Translations [Internet]. 2018 [cited 22 May 2024]. Available from: https://judithlasker.com/perinatal-grief-scale/

20. Hassan BA, Elmugabil A, Alhabrdi NA, Ahmed ABA, Rayis DA, Adam I. Maternal age and miscarriage: A unique association curve in Sudan. African Journal of Reproductive Health. 16 August 2022;26(7):15-21.

21. Chou B. The Johns Hopkins Manual of Gynecology and Obstetrics. 6th edition. Philadelphia: LWW; 2020. 856 p.

22. Gilmore J. Body mass index and health.

23. Physical status: the use of and interpretation of anthropometry, report of a WHO expert committee [Internet]. [cited 22 May 2024]. Available from: https://www.who.int/publications-detail-redirect/9241208546

24. Feodor Nilsson S, Andersen PK, Strandberg-Larsen K, Nybo Andersen AM. Risk factors for miscarriage from a prevention perspective: a nationwide follow-up study. BJOG. Oct 2014;121(11):1375-84.

25. Ghimire PR, Akombi-Inyang BJ, Tannous C, Agho KE. Association between obesity and miscarriage among women of reproductive age in Nepal. PLOS ONE. 6 August 2020;15(8):e0236435.

26. Saxov KR, Strandberg-Larsen K, Pristed SG, Bruun NH, Kesmodel US. Maternal alcohol consumption and the risk of miscarriage in the first and second trimesters: A systematic review and dose-response meta-analysis. Acta Obstetricia et Gynecologica Scandinavica. 1 Jul 2023;102(7):821-32.

27. Sundermann AC, Zhao S, Young CL, Lam L, Jones SH, Velez Edwards DR, et al. Alcohol Use in Pregnancy and Miscarriage: A Systematic Review and Meta-Analysis.

Alcoholism: Clinical and Experimental Research. 2019;43(8):1606-16.

28. Smoking and Miscarriage Risk: Epidemiology [Internet]. [cited 22 May 2024]. Available sur:
https://journals.lww.com/epidem/fulltext/2010/11000/smoking_and_miscarriage_risk.33.as px
29. Pineles BL, Park E, Samet JM. Systematic review and meta-analysis of miscarriage and maternal exposure to tobacco smoke during pregnancy. Am J Epidemiol. 1 Apr 2014;179(7):807-23.

30. Aune D, Saugstad OD, Henriksen T, Tonstad S. Maternal body mass index and the risk of fetal death, stillbirth, and infant death: a systematic review and meta-analysis. JAMA. 16 Apr 2014;311(15):1536-46.

31. Bouiller C. Couples' experiences of first trimester miscarriage. 2014 [cited 22 May 2024]; Available from: https://sonar.ch/global/documents/315236

32. Wright PM. The pushing on theory of maternal perinatal bereavement. In: Perinatal and pediatric bereavement in nursing and other health professions [Internet]. New York, NY, US: Springer Publishing Company; 2016. p. 71-96. Available from:
https://psycnet.apa.org/record/2015-50976-005

33. Emond - parents and nurses.pdf [Internet]. [cited 25 Apr 2024]. Available from:
https://corpus.ulaval.ca/server/api/core/bitstreams/3f9cb5d8-a0f8-423b-ac27-
faee9fcce682/content

34. Potvin L, Lasker J, Toedter L. Measuring grief: A short version of the Perinatal Grief Scale. Journal of Psychopathology and Behavioral Assessment. March 1, 1989;11:29-45.

35. Prommanart N, Phatharayuttawat S, Boriboonhirunsarn D, Sunsaneevithayakul P. Maternal Grief after Abortion and Related Factors. 2004;87.

36. Gozuyesil E, Manav AI, Yesilot SB, Sucu M. Grief and ruminative thought after perinatal loss among Turkish women: one-year cohort study. Sao Paulo Med J. 14 March 2022;140(2):188-98.

37. Beaudet L, Montigny F de. Lorsque la vie éclate: l'impact de la mort d'un enfant sur la famille. Paris: SeliArslan [u.a.]; 1997. 472 p.

38. Dyregrov A, Dyregrov K. Long-term impact of sudden infant death: a 12- to 15-year follow-up. Death Stud. 1999;23(7):635-61.

39. Tudehope DI, Iredell J, Rodgers D, Gunn A. Neonatal death: grieving families. Med J Aust. 17 March 1986;144(6):290-2.

40. Djiba A. A PARTIAL REQUIREMENT FOR THE MASTER'S DEGREE IN SOCIAL WORK OFFERED AT THE UNIVERSITÉ DU QUÉBEC À CHICOUTIMI UNDER A MEMORANDUM OF UNDERSTANDING WITH THE UNIVERSITÉ DU QUÉBEC EN OUTAOUAIS.

41. Tzonou A, Hsieh CC, Trichopoulos D, Aravandinos D, Kalandidi A, Margaris D, et al. Induced abortions, miscarriages, and tobacco smoking as risk factors for secondary infertility. J Epidemiol Community Health. Feb 1993;47(1):36-9.

42. Explanatory model of health in bereaved parents post-fetal/infant death | Request PDF [Internet]. [cited 22 May 2024]. Available from at: https://www.researchgate.net/publication/8238793_Explanatory_model_of_health_in_bere aved_parents_post-fetalinfant_death

43. Speraw SR. The experience of miscarriage: how couples define quality in health care delivery. J Perinatol. 1994;14(3):208-15.

44. Swanson KM, Karmali ZA, Powell SH, Pulvermakher F. Miscarriage effects on couples' interpersonal and sexual relationships during the first year after loss: women's perceptions. Psychosom Med. 2003;65(5):902-10.

45. Beutel M, Willner H, Deckardt R, Von Rad M, Weiner H. Similarities and differences in couples' grief reactions following a miscarriage: results from a longitudinal study. J Psychosom Res. March 1996;40(3):245-53.

46. Black RB. Women's voices after pregnancy loss: couples' patterns of communication and support. Soc Work Health Care. 1991;16(2):19-36.

47. Conway K, Russell G. Couples' grief and experience of support in the aftermath of miscarriage. Br J Med Psychol. Dec 2000;73 Pt 4:531-45.

48. Social and cultural factors associated with perinatal grief in Chhattisgarh, India - PubMed [Internet]. [cited 25 May 2024]. Available from: https://pubmed.ncbi.nlm.nih.gov/21956647/

49. Cohain JS, Buxbaum RE, Mankuta D. Spontaneous first trimester miscarriage rates per woman among parous women with 1 or more pregnancies of 24 weeks or more. BMC Pregnancy Childbirth. 22 Dec 2017;17(1):437.

50. Major depressive disorder in the 6 months after miscarriage - PubMed [Internet]. [cited 22 May 2024]. Available from: https://pubmed.ncbi.nlm.nih.gov/9010170/

51. Cognitive processes in psychological adaptation to miscarriage: A preliminary report. [Internet]. [cited 22 May 2024]. Available from: https://psycnet.apa.org/record/1994-18126-001

52. J. Toedter JNL Hettie JEM Janssen ,Lori. International Comparison of Studies Using the Perinatal Grief Scale: A Decade of Research on Pregnancy Loss. Death Studies. 1 Apr 2001;25(3):205-28.

53. Köneş MÖ, Yıldız H. The level of grief in women with pregnancy loss: a prospective evaluation of the first three months of perinatal loss. J Psychosom Obstet Gynaecol. dec 2021;42(4):346-55.

54. Ridaura I, Penelo E, Raich RM. Depressive symptomatology and grief in Spanish women

who have suffered a perinatal loss.

55. Yf T, Hr C, Yp C, Sf Y, Pt C. Grief reactions of couples to perinatal loss: A one-year prospective follow-up. Journal of clinical nursing [Internet]. dec 2017 [cited 22 May 2024];26(23-24). Available from: https://pubmed.ncbi.nlm.nih.gov/28880461/

56. Depressive disorder and grief following spontaneous abortion | BMC Psychiatry | Full Text [Internet]. [cited 22 May 2024]. Available from: https://bmcpsychiatry.biomedcentral.com/articles/10.1186/s12888-016-0812-y
57. Avelin P, Rådestad I, Säflund K, Wredling R, Erlandsson K. Parental grief and relationships after the loss of a stillborn baby. Midwifery. June 2013;29(6):668-73.

Appendix 1: Socio-demographic questionnaire

Ministry of Health Sfax Higher School of Health Sciences and Techniques		University of Sfax Ministry of Education Superior and of and Research Scientist

Questionnaire

In the framework of the preparation of our projectdefinstudy entitled: **"Physical and psychological impacts/repercussions of a miscarriage"**, we are asking you to answer our questionnaire as spontaneously as possible so that we can make a success of our survey. **Please note that the information and answers collected will be treated as strictly anonymous and confidential.**

Directed by : Idoudi Dhouha Hajjej Malek	National diploma in maieutic sciences / midwifery	Under the direction of : Dr. Hakim Hana Mrs Feki Khouloud

ID number:

Presentation of the woman's civil status

1) How old are you? years old

2) Where do you come from?

3)) Marital status: ☐ Married ☐ Single ☐ Divorced ☐ Widowed.

4) Level of education: ☐ Not enrolled ☐ Primary ☐ Secondary ☐ University/higher

5)Profession :

7)Socio-economic level: ☐ Low ☐ Medium☐ High

Health and lifestyle

8)Size cmWeight kg
9) Do you drink alcohol?
☐ Yes ☐ No
10)Are you a smoker?
☐ No, I've never smoked
☐ No, I don't smoke at the moment; I stopped over a year ago.
☐ Yes, I sometimes smoke (less than one cigarette a day)
☐ Yes, I smoke regularly (between 1 and 9 cigarettes a day)
☐ Yes, I smoke regularly (more than 10 cigarettes a day)
11)Personal medical history : ☐ Yes ☐ No

If yes, please specify /

12)Surgical history: ☐ Yes ☐ No

If yes, please specify //

Questions about fertility

14)Have you **tried** to get pregnant for more than a year?☐ No☐Yes

14a) Gestité (Total number of pregnancies you have had, including those that did not result in a live birth.) : //

14b) Parity (Total number of births you have had, excluding pregnancies that did not result in a live birth): //

14c) Number of living children, How many children do you have?//

14d) Number of children deceased: //

16) Number of caesarean sections: //

17) Have you ever had a miscarriage?☐ No ☐Yes

17a) If "Yes", how many times: / /

17b) Year of miscarriage(s)://

17c)Lost pregnancy is: induced ☐spontaneous☐

If induced:IVF ☐ ICSI ☐ Induction of ovulation☐

17d) At what stage of pregnancy did the miscarriage(s) occur?

First miscarriage	Before week 12 ☐	After the week 12 ☐	Complete spontaneous abortion☐	Incomplete abortion curetage	follo w-up	fro m
Second miscarriage	Before week 12 ☐	After the week 12 ☐	Complete spontaneous abortion☐	Incomplete abortion curettage	follo w-up	fro m
Third miscarriage	Before week 12 ☐	After the week 12 ☐				
Fourth miscarriage	Before week 12 ☐	After the week 12 ☐	Complete spontaneous abortion☐	Incomplete abortion curettage	follo w-up	fro m
Fifth miscarriage	Before week 12 ☐	After the week 12 ☐				
Sixth miscarriage	Before week 12 ☐	After the week 12 ☐	Complete spontaneous abortion☐	Incomplete abortion curettage	follo w-up	fro m
Seventh miscarriage	Before week 12 ☐	After the week 12 ☐				
Eighth miscarriage	Before week 12 ☐	After the week 12 ☐	Complete spontaneous abortion☐	Incomplete abortion curettage	follo w-up	fro m

18) What physical symptoms did you experience that led you to seek medical advice during your miscarriage? (Choose all that apply) :

Heavy bleeding☐Slight bleeding ☐Uterine contractions ☐No noticeable physical symptoms

Discovered during medical consultation☐ (please specify):

Followed by : // 1 = Gynaecologist; 2 = Doctor; 3 = Midwife; 4 = Matron

Questions about miscarriage / Psychological impact

19) Do you feel that you were adequately supported by the professionals looking after you?

☐ Fully supported; ☐ Supported to some extent; ☐ Not sufficiently supported; ☐ Not at all supported
20) Have you used psychological support? ☐ No☐Yes
20a) If yes, please specify the type of psychological support :
☐ Individual follow-up with a psychologist
☐ Mari
☐ Friends
☐ Family support
☐ Other (please specify):
21) How would you describe your partner's reaction to the situation?
☐ Emotionally affected and sad; ☐ Expressing feelings of guilt or blame;

Supportive and understanding; ☐ Passive and withdrawn; ☐ Other (specify):
22) Did you develop a bad impression of the hospital as a result of this experience? ☐ No ☐Yes
23) What is the estimated duration of these feelings?
Less than 3 months ☐ 3-6 months;☐ More than 6 months
24) Did you notice any signs of vaginismus after the miscarriage? ☐ No ☐Yes
25) Have you experienced vaginismus (an involuntary contraction of the vaginal muscles, leading to difficulty or impossibility of penetration), since the miscarriage? ☐ No ☐Yes

26) Reduced sleep
Represents the experience of a reduction in the duration or depth of sleep compared with the subject's usual pattern when in good health.
☐ Asleep as usual
☐ Slight difficulty in falling asleep or slightly reduced, light or restless sleep.
☐ Reduced or interrupted sleep of at least two hours.
☐ Less than two or three hours' sleep.
27) Reduced appetite
Represents the sensation of loss of appetite compared with the normal state. Assess the loss of desire to eat or the need to force yourself to eat.

☐   Normal or increased appetite

☐ Slightly reduced appetite.

☐ No appetite. The food is bland.

☐ Need persuasion/encouragement to eat.

28) Difficulty concentrating

Difficulty gathering thoughts, which can lead to a lack of concentration. Assess according to intensity, frequency and degree of disability.

☐ No concentration difficulties

☐ Occasional difficulty gathering thoughts.

☐ Difficulty concentrating and thinking straight, which reduces the ability to read or hold a conversation.

☐ Inability to read or express without great difficulty.

Physical impact

29) Do you have any concerns about meeting

Difficulties conceiving following your abortion? ☐ No☐Yes

30) Have you consulted or are you considering consulting a healthcare professional to deal with any problems related to post-abortive infertility? ☐ No ☐Yes

31) Have you experienced any of the following complications since your miscarriage?

Fever☐ No☐Yes

Pelvic pain☐ No☐Yes

Lochies with a foul odour☐ No☐Yes

Profuse and purulent vaginal discharge☐ No☐Yes

III. The impact of miscarriage on a woman's relationship with her partner

32) How would you assess your relationship with your husband after the miscarriage?

Unchanged ☐ ; Improvement ☐ ; Degradation ☐

Ifimprovement or deterioration, please explain briefly the perceived changes:

33) With regard to your sexual life after the miscarriage, how did you feel and experience intimate relations?

☐ Feeling of obligation (If you felt pressure or a duty to maintain sexual activity)

☐ Unchanged (If your sex life has remained similar to before the miscarriage)

☐ Fear of another pregnancy (If the fear of another pregnancy has influenced your sex life)

☐ No sexuality (if you have chosen to abstain or if the miscarriage has negatively affected your intimacy)

Appendix 2

	Strongly Agree	Agree	Neither Agree nor Disagree	Disagree	Strongly Disagree
1. I feel depressed.	1	2	3	4	5
2. I find it hard to get along with certain people.	1	2	3	4	5
3. I feel empty inside.	1	2	3	4	5
4. I can't keep up with my normal activities.	1	2	3	4	5
5. I feel a need to talk about the baby.	1	2	3	4	5
6. I am grieving for the baby.	1	2	3	4	5
7. I am frightened.	1	2	3	4	5
8. I have considered suicide since the loss.	1	2	3	4	5
9. I take medicine for my nerves.	1	2	3	4	5
10. I very much miss the baby.	1	2	3	4	5
11. I feel I have adjusted well to the loss.	1	2	3	4	5
12. It is painful to recall memories of the loss.	1	2	3	4	5
13. I get upset when I think about the baby.	1	2	3	4	5

	Strongly Agree	Agree	Neither Agree nor Disagree	Disagree	Strongly Disagree
14. I cry when I think about him/her.	1	2	3	4	5
15. I feel guilty when I think about the baby.	1	2	3	4	5
16. I feel physically ill when I think about the baby.	1	2	3	4	5
17. I feel unprotected in a dangerous world since he/she died.	1	2	3	4	5

	Agree	Disagree	Disagree	Strongly Disagree
18. I try to laugh, but 1 nothing seems funny anymore.	2	3	4	5
19. Time passes so slowly 1 since the baby died.	2	3	4	5
20. The best part of me died 1 2 with the baby.	3		4	5
21. I have let people down 1 2 since the baby died.	3		4	5
22. I feel worthless since 1 2 he/she died.	3		4	5
23. I blame myself for the 1 2 baby's death.	3		4	5
24. I get cross at my 1 2 friends and relatives more than I should.	3		4	5
25. Sometimes I feel like I 2 1 need a professional counselor to help me get my life back together again .	3		4	5

Strongly Agree	Agree	Neither Agree nor Disagree	Disagree	Strongly Disagree
26. I feel as though I'm just 1 existing and not really living since he/she died.	2	3	4	5
27. I feel so lonely since 1 he/she died.	2	3	4	5
28. I feel somewhat apart and 1 remote, even among friends.	2	3	4	5
29. It's safer not to love. 1	2	3	4	5
30. I find it difficult to 1 make decisions since the baby died.	2	3	4	5
31. I worry about what my 1 future will be like.	2	3	4	5
32. Being a bereaved parent 1 means being a "Second- Class Citizen".	2	3	4	5
33. It feels great to be alive. 1	2	3	4	5

SUMMARY

Introduction: *Emerging evidence suggests that miscarriage is associated with significant and potentially long-lasting psychological and physical consequences. Despite the high frequency of pregnancies complicated by miscarriage, there are no available data on the psychological impacts, particularly perinatal bereavement, as well as the possible physical impacts in Tunisian women who have experienced a miscarriage.*

Material and methods: *We conducted a descriptive and analytical study. It took place mainly in the obstetrics and gynaecology department of the CHU Hédi Chaker in Sfax, including the postpartum, gynaecology and high-risk pregnancy departments, as well as outpatient consultations, during the period from 12 February to 31 March 2024. Data were collected using a sociodemographic, obstetric and gynaecological data collection form and the PGS-33 perinatal bereavement scale. The main objective of this research is to describe the physical and psychological consequences of miscarriage for Tunisian women.*

Results: The *average age of the women in our population was 32, 40.4% had secondary education and 57.8% were multiparous. As for the number of living children, 55% of the women had between 2 and 4 children. The mean PGS score was 103.57, with a significant standard deviation of 27.17, with 67.9% of women having total scores above or equal to the threshold (≥ 91). In terms of physical repercussions, 69.7% reported difficulty in falling asleep, 67.9% reported a disturbance in their appetite, and 44% reported post-abortive vaginismus. A statistically significant difference was found between the mean values of the PGS total score in terms of the "origin" variable (P= 0.029 < 0,05). No statistically significant difference was found with age and occupational status (P= 0.334 and P= 0.160, respectively). Similarly, a significant difference was found between the mean values of the PGS total score in terms of the number of HRs ($\chi2= 7.82$; P=0.020).*

Conclusion: *A holistic approach incorporating psychological and physical care is essential to help women overcome the grief associated with miscarriage.*

Key word : *Miscarriage - Psychological impact - Perinatal bereavement - Physical impact*

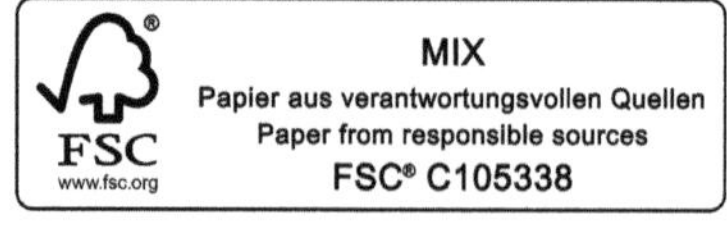

Printed by Books on Demand GmbH, Norderstedt / Germany